Needling
Techniques
for
Acupuncturists

of related interest

Tuina / Massage Manipulations
Basic Principles and Techniques
Editor in Chief: Li Jiangshan
ISBN 978 1 84819 058 0

Illustrated Treatment for Migraine using Acupuncture, Moxibustion and Tuina Massage
Cui Chengbin and Xing Xiaomin
ISBN 978 1 84819 061 0

Illustrated Treatment for Cervical Spondylosis Using Massage
Tang Xuezhang and Yu Tianyuan
ISBN 978 1 84819 062 7

Meridians and Acupoints
Edited by Zhu Bing and Wang Hongcai
Advisor: Cheng Xinnong
ISBN 978 1 84819 037 5

Basic Theories of Traditional Chinese Medicine
Edited by Zhu Bing and Wang Hongcai
Advisor: Cheng Xinnong
ISBN 978 1 84819 038 2

Acupuncture Therapeutics
Edited by Zhu Bing and Wang Hongcai
Advisor: Cheng Xinnong
ISBN 978 1 84819 039 9

Diagnostics of Traditional Chinese Medicine
Edited by Zhu Bing and Wang Hongcai
Advisor: Cheng Xinnong
ISBN 978 1 84819 036 8

Case Studies from the Medical Records of Leading Chinese Acupuncture Experts
Edited by Zhu Bing and Wang Hongcai
Advisor: Cheng Xinnong
ISBN 978 1 84819 046 7

Needling
Techniques
for
Acupuncturists

Basic Principles and Techniques

Chief Editor: Professor Chang Xiaorong

SINGING
DRAGON

LONDON AND PHILADELPHIA

Translators: Yang Qianyun, Lan Lei and Chen Huachu
Assistant Editors: Yuan Yiqin and Ai'kun
Editorial Committee: Yang Qianyun, Wang Chao, Lan Lei and Guo Tingxiang

First published in 2009
by People's Military Medical Press

This edition published in 2011
by Singing Dragon
an imprint of Jessica Kingsley Publishers
in co-operation with People's Military Medical Press
116 Pentonville Road
London N1 9JB, UK
and
400 Market Street, Suite 400
Philadelphia, PA 19106, USA

www.singingdragon.com

Library of Congress Cataloging in Publication Data
A CIP catalog record for this book is available from the Library of Congress

British Library Cataloguing in Publication Data
A CIP catalogue record for this book is available from the British Library

ISBN 978 1 84819 057 3

Printed and Bound in Great Britain by
MPG Books Group

Contents

Introduction

This book is written for TCM (Traditional Chinese Medicine) college acupuncture students, and primary medical personnel. The book is divided into 11 chapters with an introduction on the structure and specifications of the filiform needle, and how to maintain it; needling practices; preparations; methods of insertion; direction, angle and depth of insertion; manipulations and the arrival of *qi*; the reinforcing and reducing methods of acupuncture; four comprehensive needling manipulations called Dragon–Tiger–Tortoise–Phoenix (*Fei Jing Zou Qi Si Fa*); retention and withdrawal of needles; management and prevention of accidents; precautions, etc. Practice essentials and manipulation of the needling techniques are described with both pictures and text in order to make the subject as clear as possible for readers. The book is easy to understand and a DVD demonstrating the needling techniques is also provided for ease of learning.

CHAPTER 1

Structure, Specification, Checking and Maintenance of the Filiform Needle

1. Structure of the Filiform Needle

Filiform needles are made of metal. They are usually made of stainless steel and nowadays widely used in clinic because of their high strength and toughness, straight and smooth shape, and resistance to high temperature, rustiness and chemicals. (Fig. 1)

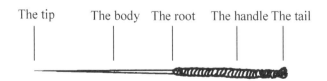

Fig. 1 Structure of the filiform needle

A filiform needle is divided into five parts: the tip, the body, the root, the handle and the tail.

- *The tip (zhen mang)* is the sharp point of the needle, it is the key part of the needle that is punctured through the skin.

- *The body (zhen ti)* is the main part between the tip and the handle; it is the main part that is inserted to the appropriate depth in the acupoint.

- *The root* connects the body and the handle, and is the external sign to indicate the puncturing depth of the body and the range of lifting and thrusting.

- *The handle* is the part of the needle from the root to the tail and it is usually wrapped in a helical style with metal wire; it is the place where the practitioner holds and manipulates the needle, as well as the location for fixing moxa in warming acupuncture.

- *The tail (zhen ding)* is the end of the handle.

2. Specification of the Filiform Needle

Specifications of filiform needles are distinguished by the diameter and length of the body. See Table 1 and Table 2 below. No. 28–30 (0.32–0.38mm) and 1–3 *cun* (25–75mm) filiform needles are most commonly used in clinic.

Ling-shu Guan-zhen points out: 'Nine kinds of needles are appropriate to different conditions. The sizes and lengths of them are also different. You can use them to remove diseases.' That is to say, each different needle has its respective characters and effects; corresponding needles can be chosen to treat different symptoms. Needles of different specification can be chosen in clinic according to the constitution, body shape, age, condition and acupoint position of the patients.

Table 1 Lengths of Filiform Needles

Cun[1]	0.5	1.0	1.5	2.0	2.5	3.0	3.5	4.0	4.5
Length (mm)	15	25	40	50	65	75	90	100	115

Table 2 Diameters of Filiform Needles

No.	26	27	28	29	30	31	32	33
Diameter (mm)	0.45	0.42	0.38	0.34	0.32	0.30	0.28	0.26

3. Checking the Filiform Needle

Check carefully before and after use. Damaged needles must be removed and repaired before they are used.

3.1 Checking the Tip

You can hold the handle and twirl it with your thumb, forefinger and middle finger while touching the tip with the third finger of the same hand so that you can check the tip and see whether it is curled or hooked. You can also use an

---

1   Cun is a Chinese unit of length. 1 cun = 3.33cm.

alcohol-soaked cotton ball to wrap the lower segment of the disinfected needle body with your left hand; hold the handle with one hand; then repeatedly rotate the tip in the cotton ball and withdraw it. If the needle is found to be unsmooth or there is cotton left attached to it, it is hooked.

3.2 Checking the Body

We can make a visual inspection to see whether the body is obviously bent or eroded. If it does not appear bent, place it flat on the table and roll it through 360° slowly. If the body keeps flat on the table all the time, it is not bent; on the other hand, if some part of the body doesn't stay flat on the table and is lifted up like an arch when rolling, this part is bent. The degree of the bend and the height of the arch are directly proportional. The higher the arch, the more bent the body.

4. Taking Care of the Filiform Needle

The maintenance of reusable needles should be paid attention to, and of course this is not necessary for disposable needles. In order to prevent damage to the tips and bending, rust, or contamination of the bodies, the needles should be kept properly. Needles are usually kept in the needle boxes, tubes and bags. Needle boxes or bags should be padded and covered with some sterile gauzes to prevent contamination. Disinfected needles should be put on or inserted in the sterile gauze according to their lengths, and finally the needle boxes or the needle bags are closed for later applications.

CHAPTER 2

Needling Practice

Needling practice mainly involves building up good finger force and developing skill in manipulation. Practitioners must practice frequently to develop finger force and ability to manipulate the needle until they become skilful and able to insert a needle swiftly through the skin without causing pain, as well as freely manipulating the needle for reinforcing and reducing. Otherwise, with unskilled finger force and manipulation, practitioners will have difficulty in inserting and controlling the needles and this will cause obvious pain and feel awkward when manipulating. Needling practice is generally carried out in three steps.

1. Finger Force Practice

Fold soft paper into a small paper cushion about 8cm × 5cm across and 2–3cm thick, then bind the cushion like '井' with thread. When practicing, hold the paper cushion in the left hand and hold the needle handle with the right thumb, index and middle finger; hold the 1–1.5 *cun* needle firmly but with a loose wrist and hold it vertically to let the tip reach the paper cushion, then twirl the needle with the right thumb, alternately with the right index and middle finger, gradually increasing the pressure till the needle penetrates the paper; then turn to another position. Practice repeatedly. Paper cushion practice is the basic method to develop finger force and twirling–rotating manipulation. (Fig. 2)

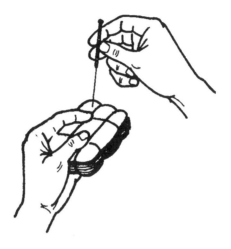

Fig. 2 Finger force practice

2. Manipulation Practice

Manipulation practice is usually carried out with a cotton ball. Get some cotton, wind it with thread to make a cotton ball about 6–7cm in diameter, dense outside and loose inside; then wrap it with a piece of cloth and sew it thoroughly. As the cotton ball is soft, various manipulations such as lifting and thrusting, twirling and rotating, as well as inserting and withdrawing can be imitated and practiced. When practicing lifting–thrusting, hold the needle tight but with a loose wrist; insert it into the cotton ball and make lifting and thrusting movement in the same place with appropriate depth and even amplitude. The needle body should be kept perpendicular. (Fig. 3)

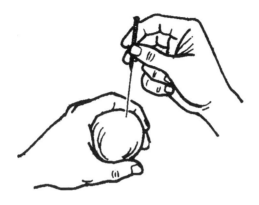

Fig. 3 Manipulation practice

3. Needling Practice on a Body

You should practice on yourself (but only after you have developed good finger force and skilful manipulations by practicing on the paper cushion and cotton ball) so that you can gain personal experiences of feeling finger force and needling sensations and can practice manipulations. You should gradually try to obtain painless, perpendicular, smooth insertions and manipulate smooth lifting and thrusting, twirling and rotating with even finger force and skilful manipulation.

CHAPTER 3

Preparation

1. Selection of the Filiform Needles

Selection of the filiform needles is based on sex, age, physique and constitution; the nature of disease; the interior or exterior location of the disease; and the location of the acupoints. For example, we use longer and larger filiform needles on male patients who are strong, fat, and whose diseases are much deeper. We use shorter and smaller filiform needles on female patients who are weak, thin, and whose diseases are more superficial. As far as selection according to the location of the acupoints, longer, thicker filiform needles are usually used on the areas with thick muscles and skin and are appropriate for deep needling; shorter, thinner filiform needles are used on the areas with thin muscles and skins and are appropriate for shallow needling. We should insert the needle to the right depth with some part of the body of the needle outside the skin. For example, we should use a 1.0 *cun* filiform needle to insert an acupoint 0.5 *cun*, and use a 1.5–2.0 *cun* filiform needle to insert an acupoint 1.0 *cun*.

2. Postural Alignment and Positioning

The position of the patient's body is important for the correct location of acupoints, correct manipulation, and prolonged retention of the needle; it is also important for prevention of fainting during needle insertion, stuck needles, bent needles and broken needles. For example, if a weak patient with a serious disease or a nervous patient adopts a sitting position, he easily starts to feel fatigue and is prone to fainting. The commonly-used needling positions and postures in clinic are as follows.

2.1 Supine Position (Lying on the Back)

This position is suitable for acupoints on the head, face, nape, chest, abdomen and limbs. (Fig. 4)

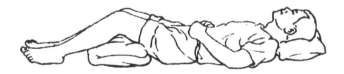

Fig. 4 Lying on the back

2.2 Lateral Recumbent Position (Lying on the Side)

This position is suitable for the acupoints of Shaoyang Meridian on the lateral side of the body and some acupoints on the arms and legs. (Fig. 5)

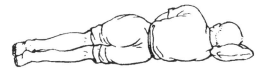

Fig. 5 Lying on the side

2.3 Prone Position (Lying on the Belly)

This position is suitable for acupoints on the head, nape, shoulder, back, lumbar and buttock regions and the posterior region of the lower limbs and some acupoints on the upper limbs. (Fig. 6)

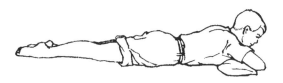

Fig. 6 Lying on the belly

2.4 Supine Sitting Position

This position is suitable for the acupoints on the forehead, face and nape. (Fig. 7)

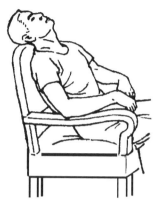

Fig. 7 Supine sitting

2.5 Prone Sitting Position

This position is suitable for the acupoints of the occiput, nape and back. (Fig. 8)

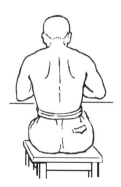

Fig. 8 Prone sitting

2.6 Lateral Prone Sitting Position

This position is suitable for the acupoints of the lateral sides of the head, cheeks and ears. (Fig. 9)

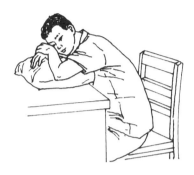

Fig. 9 Lateral prone sitting

3. Disinfection

Strict aseptic technique must be faithfully adhered to throughout every treatment so as to avoid unnecessary infection. The following things should be disinfected before needling: needles and needling apparatus, both hands of the practitioner, the patient's manipulation position and the appliances in the medical treatment room.

3.1 Disinfection of Needles and Needling Apparatus

There are many disinfection methods for needles and needling apparatus. The best one is autoclave sterilization.

1. *Autoclave sterilization:* Needles wrapped in cloth should be sterilized in an autoclave at 1.0–1.4 kg/cm² and

115–123°C for 30 minutes to satisfy the requirements of sterilization.

2. *Chemical disinfection*: Needles should be placed into a 75% solution of alcohol for 30–60 minutes, then they should be taken out and wiped off with a sterile towel or sterile cotton ball before use. Needles can also be put into a disinfectant such as '84' solution (sodium hypochlorite, or bleach) and can be disinfected according to the specified concentration and time. Appliances which are in direct contact with the filiform needles, such as needle trays, tubes, boxes and tweezers can also be put into a disinfectant such as 2% lysol solution or 1:1000 mercuric chloride solution for 1–2 hours and can be used after meeting the requirements of disinfection. Disinfected needles should be put in disinfected needle trays and covered with a sterile towel or sterile gauzes.

3. *Boiling*: Needles and other apparatus wrapped in cloth can be disinfected in boiled water for 15–20 min. However, it should be noted that boiling can blunt the sharp metal appliance. If 2% Sodium Bicarbonate is added, this can raise the boiling point to 120°C and prevent corrosion.

3.2 Finger Disinfection

Practitioners should wash and brush their hands and fingernails with soap and water before needling. After their hands are dry, wipe the hands with cotton balls soaked in a 75% solution of alcohol.

3.3 Skin Disinfection

Disinfect the needling position skin with cotton balls soaked in 75% solution of alcohol, or first wipe with a 2% tincture of iodine, when it is somewhat dry, next wipe with 75% alcohol cotton balls to remove the iodine. When wiping the skin, one should start from the centre of the position and continue by circling from the centre to the outer ring.

CHAPTER 4

Insertions

Both the practitioner's hands should cooperate and work closely together when needling. *Nan-jing Qi-shi-ba-nan*[1] says: 'Those who know a lot about acupuncture believe in their left hands, while the ones who do not, believe only in their right hands.' *Biao You Fu*[2] explains: 'Press heavily with the left hand several times, so as to let *qi* disperse; insert slowly and lightly with the right hand so as to cause no pain.' Usually the right hand is used for holding the needle, and mainly holds the handle of a needle with the thumb and index finger, or the thumb, index finger and the middle finger, with the needle held vertical (Fig. 10), so the right hand is called the 'puncturing (needling) hand'. The left hand that assists or presses the body part is called the 'pressing (palpating) hand'.

---

1   *Nan-jing* is a classic Chinese medicine textbook, explaining 81 important theories in question and answer format. *Qi-shi-ba-nan* is question number 78.
2   *Biao You Fu* is an important classic textbook on acupuncture.

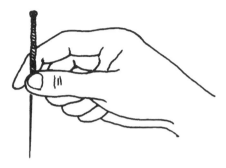

Fig. 10A Holding the needle with the thumb and index finger

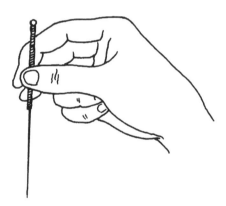

Fig. 10B Holding the needle with the thumb and middle finger

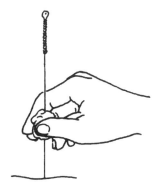

Fig. 10C Holding the body

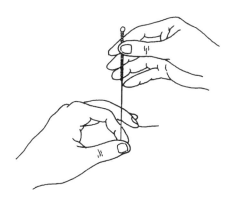

Fig. 10D Holding the needle with both hands

- *The function of the puncturing hand* is to hold the needle and to perform manipulations. During insertion, the puncturing hand generates focused force on the tip of the needle to make it penetrate the skin. During manipulation, it manipulates twirling–rotating to the left and to the right, lifting–thrusting upward and downward, plucking, trembling, scraping and rubbing. The practitioner can use some techniques during withdrawal too (e.g. see techniques on p.78).

- *The function of the pressing hand* is to fix the location of a point and to grip the needle body to help the puncturing hand to insert the needle. It can support the body of the needle, keep it straight and focus the strength directly to the tip of the needle so as to insert smoothly with less pain and facilitate the regulation and control of the needling sensations. Specific insertions used in clinic are the following.

1. Single-Handed Insertions

This method is mainly suitable for the insertion of short needles. The body of the needle is grasped with the thumb and index finger, with the pad of the middle finger approximately supporting the middle of the needle body. While pushing down with the thumb and index finger, the middle finger is flexed and inserts the needle to the appropriate depth. Since all three fingers are used in this method, it is especially applicable for doing insertions into two points simultaneously. (Fig. 11)

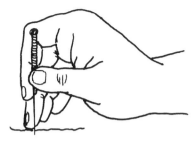

Fig. 11 Single-handed insertion

2. Double-Handed Insertions

2.1 Fingernail-Pressing Needle Insertion

Press the acupuncture point with the thumbnail or the index finger of the left hand and keep the needle tip closely to the nail, then insert the needle in the point (Fig. 12). This method is suitable for short needles.

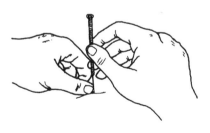

Fig. 12 Fingernail-pressing needle insertion

2.2 Hand-Holding Needle Insertion

Hold a dry sterile cotton ball around the needle tip with the thumb and index finger of the pressing hand and fix the needle tip directly over the selected point. Twirl the needle handle with the puncturing hand and insert it into the point. This method is suitable for long needles. (Fig. 13)

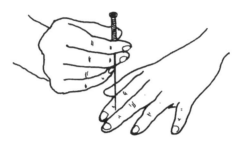

Fig. 13 Hand-holding needle insertion

2.3 Skin-Spreading Needle Insertion

Put the thumb and index fingers of the pressing hand on the skin and separate the two fingers to tautly stretch the skin. Hold the needle with the puncturing hand and insert the needle into the point through the space between the two fingers. This method is suitable for needling acupoints on positions where the skin is loose. (Fig. 14)

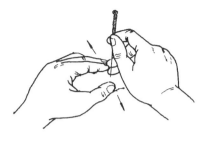

Fig. 14 Skin-spreading needle insertion

2.4 Pinching Insertion Method

Pinch the skin up around the point with the thumb and index fingers of the pressing hand. Hold the needle with the puncturing hand and insert the needle into the point in the pinched skin. This method is suitable for puncturing acupoints on positions where the muscle and skin is thin, such as Yintang (EX-HN3). (Fig. 15)

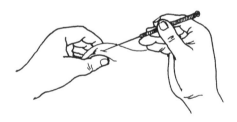

Fig. 15 Pinching insertion method

3. Point Penetration Method

The point penetration method is also called 'jointed puncture' (*Tou Zhen fa*) or 'penetration needling' (*Tou Ci fa*). In this method the practitioner inserts the needle along the skin, or inserts the needle deeply and uprightly, making the needle penetrate from one acupoint to another acupoint, playing the role of one needle with two acupoints or one needle with many acupoints. It amplifies the indications and needling sensation, and makes it easy to spread and transmit the needling sensation and let it arrive at the sick place directly so as to increase the therapeutic effect. The commonly-used penetration methods are the following two.

3.1 Penetration Needling Along the Skin

At first insert the needle at one acupoint, then let the tip aim towards another acupoint nearby; next penetrate along the skin, thus making one needle penetrate two acupoints or even three acupoints, such as penetration from Dicang (ST4) to Jiache (ST6), penetration from Yingxiang (LI20) to Sibai (ST2), penetration from Cuanzhu (BL2) to Yuyao (EX-HN4), penetration from Sizhukong (SJ23) to Shuaigu (GB8), penetration from Pishu (BL20) to Weishu (BL21), penetration from Zhongwan (RN12) to Jianli (RN11) to Xiawan (RN10). It is applicable to the acupoints of the head, face, back and abdomen. Generally the tip does not come out of the skin. (Fig. 16)

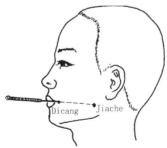

Fig. 16 Penetration from Dicang (ST4) to Jiache (ST6)

3.2 Penetration Needling Along the Gap

Penetrate the needle to the appropriate acupoint in another side along the tissue space after inserting the needle in one acupoint from one side, such as penetration from Yinlingquan (SP9) to Yanglingquan (GB34), penetration from Jianshi (PC5) to Zhigou (SJ6), penetration from Waiguan (SJ5) to Neiguan (PC6), penetration from Hegu (LI4) to Laogong (PC8). It is applicable to the acupoints on the extremities. The tip can come out of the skin. (Fig. 17)

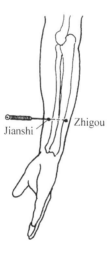

Fig. 17 Penetration from Jianshi (PC5) to Zhigou (SJ6)

4. Needle in Tube Insertions

Put the needle into a glass, plastic or metal tube (note: the tube should be shorter than the needle by about 2–3 *fen*[3] in length) and put them on the skin where the point is located. Press the tube with the pressing hand; tap the needle's tail swiftly with index finger of the puncturing hand to insert the tip of needle into the skin. Remove the tube over the needle and insert the needle into the point to the appropriate depth. (Fig. 18)

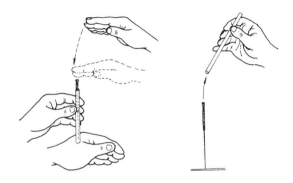

Fig. 18 Needle in tube insertion

---

3   *Fen* is a Chinese unit of length. 1 *fen* = 0.33cm.

CHAPTER 5

Direction, Angle and Depth of Insertion

Angle, direction and depth of insertion mean the specific manipulation requirements after the needle has been inserted into the skin. During the process of insertion, these aspects are especially important in acupuncture. The correct angle, direction and depth help to induce needling sensations, bring about the desired therapeutic results and guarantee safety. They are decided according to specific acupoint location, the physical condition of a patient, the nature of an illness and needling manipulations.

1. Direction of Insertion

The direction of insertion refers to the direction of the needle tip during acupuncture. Generally, it is decided according to the direction of the meridian running course, the location of a point and the desired therapeutic requirements.

1.1 According to the Running Course of the Meridian

In order to achieve the purpose of 'Ying-sui reinforcing and reducing', the practitioner should needle according to the direction of the meridian running course. Generally, needling with the tip towards the direction of the meridian running course manipulates reinforcing, and against the direction manipulates reducing.

1.2 According to the Location of the Acupoint

Deciding the direction of insertion according to the location of acupoints ensures safety when needling. For instance, the needle should be inserted slowly with the tip pointing to the direction of the mandible when needling Yamen (GV15), and slowly with the tip pointing to the direction of the tongue root when needling Lianquan (CV23), the tip should point towards the spinal column when needling some acupoints on the back.

1.3 According to the Patient's Condition

In order to make the needling sensation transmit to the diseased region, the tip should point to it or 'to promote the movement of the meridian qi to reach the diseased area'. The direction of insertion can be decided according to the patient's condition when manipulating.

2. Angle of Insertion

The angle of insertion is formed by the needle and the surface of the skin as the needle is inserted (Fig. 19). It is decided in consideration of both the location of the point and the practitioner's purpose. Generally, there are three options.

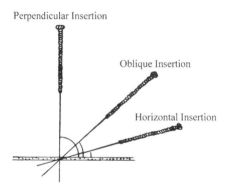

Fig. 19 Angle of insertion

2.1 Perpendicular Insertion

In this method, the needle is inserted perpendicularly, forming a 90° angle with the skin. Most points on the body can be punctured in this way.

2.2 Oblique Insertion

The needle is inserted obliquely to form an angle of approximately 45° with the skin. It is suitable for the points where the muscle is thin or close to the important viscera. Acupoints on the chest and back are often needled in this way.

2.3 Horizontal Insertion (also known as Transverse Insertion)

The needle is inserted horizontally to form a 15–25° angle with the skin. This method is commonly used in the places where the muscle is thin.

3. Depth of Needle Insertion

Clinically, the depth of insertion is also determined by the constitution, age, condition of the patient and the location of the acupoint. (Fig. 20)

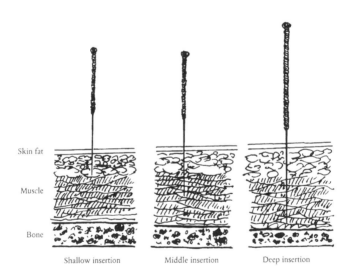

Skin fat	
Muscle	
Bone	
	Shallow insertion Middle insertion Deep insertion

Fig. 20 Depth of needle insertion

3.1 Age

Elderly patients often suffer from *qi* and blood deficiencies and infants have delicate constitutions, so deep insertions are inadvisable. However, young and middle-aged patients who are strong can be given deep insertions.

3.2 The Constitution of the Patient

Relatively shallow insertions should be done on lean, weak patients, and deep insertions on strong, robust patients.

3.3 The Patient's Condition

Yang syndromes and acute diseases should be treated with shallow insertions; while *Yin* syndromes and chronic diseases with deep insertions.

3.4 The Location of the Points

Points on the head and face, chest and belly, and areas where the skins and muscles are thin should be given shallow insertions.

CHAPTER 6

Manipulations and Arrival of *Qi* (Needling Sensation)

Manipulations, also known as needling transmissions, are methods of operation designed to produce needling sensation for the patients, and to adjust the sensation so as to transmit the sensation in a specific direction. Generally, manipulation techniques can be divided into two categories: fundamental and auxiliary.

1. The Fundamental Manipulation Techniques

The fundamental manipulations refer to the basic operation methods with filiform needles. Those most commonly used are lifting–thrusting and twirling–rotating. These two basic techniques can either be used separately or in conjunction with each other.

1.1 Lifting and Thrusting

This is a method of operation in which the manipulation involves rising upward and inserting downward after inserting the needle to a certain depth. Thrusting refers to inserting the needle from the superficial layer down to the deep layer. Lifting means withdrawal of the needle from the deep layer up to the superficial layer. The above mentioned repeated vertical up and down movement is known as lifting and thrusting. The extent of up and down movement should be moderate, about 3–5 *fen* in depth; the frequency should also be moderate at about 60 times every minute. Be sure to keep the needle straight to avoid changing its angle and direction. Generally, lifting and thrusting to a large degree and at a high frequency may induce a strong stimulation, and to a small degree and at a low frequency lead to a weak stimulation. (Fig. 21)

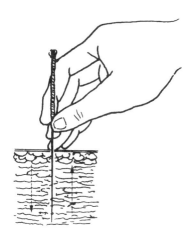

Fig. 21 Lifting and thrusting

1.2 Twirling and Rotating

This is a method of operation in which the manipulation involves twirling and rotating the needle forward and backward after inserting it to a certain depth. In other words, the repeated forward and backward rotation movement is called twirling and rotating (Fig. 22). The amplitude, frequency and duration of the manipulation depend on the constitution and condition of the patient, the location of the acupoint, and the purpose of acupuncture. Finger force should be even during the manipulation, and the amplitude should be moderate at about 180–360°. Unidirectional twirling should not be done; otherwise the muscle fibre can wrap in the body and lead to local pain and stuck needles or even difficult withdrawal. Generally, lifting and thrusting to a large degree and at a high frequency may induce a strong stimulation, and to a small degree and at a low frequency lead to a weak stimulation.

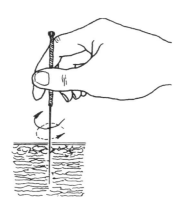

Fig. 22 Twirling and rotating

2. Auxiliary Techniques

The auxiliary techniques are supplements to the fundamental ones for the purpose of promoting the arrival of meridian *qi* and enhancing needling sensation. Those commonly used in the clinic are as follows.

2.1 Pressing

If *qi* doesn't arrive, pressing can be used to promote *qi*. Slightly press the skin along the course of the meridian to encourage the movement of *qi* and blood and stimulate meridian *qi*. (Fig. 23)

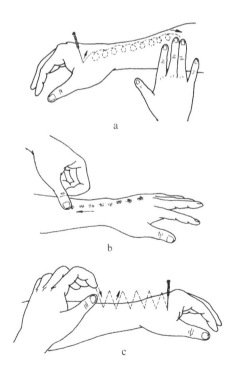

a

b

c

Fig. 23 Pressing

2.2 Plucking

Pluck the handle of the needle lightly and make it tremble in order to enhance the needling sensation and circulate *qi*. This is used for promoting and stimulating *qi*. (Fig. 24)

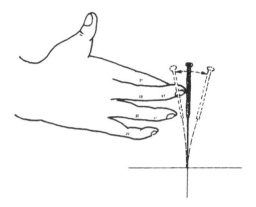

Fig. 24 Plucking

2.3 Scraping

If the needle is inserted and *qi* doesn't arrive, place the thumb (the index finger or the middle finger) of the right hand on the tail end to keep the needle steady, scrape the handle repeatedly with the nail of the index finger (the middle finger or the thumb) of the right hand upward or downward for promoting *qi*. After *qi* arrives, it can strengthen the transmission and spread of the needling sensation. (Fig. 25)

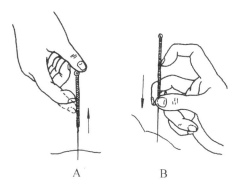

Fig. 25 Scraping

2.4 Shaking

After inserting the needle to a certain depth, hold the handle and shake the body to promote the circulation of *qi*. There are two ways of shaking. One is shaking with the body upright to promote the needling sensation; the other is shaking with the body transverse to transmit the meridian *qi* to a certain direction. (Fig. 26)

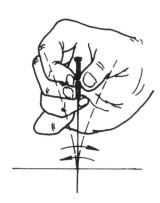

Fig. 26 Shaking

2.5 Flying

Twirl the needle several times, and then suddenly release and separate the thumb and the index finger from it, do twirling and releasing repeatedly. The movement looks like a bird spreading its wings to fly, so it is termed flying. Flying can promote and circulate *qi*, as well as strengthen the needling sensation. (Fig. 27)

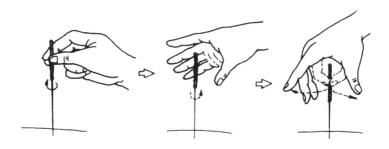

Fig. 27 Flying

2.6 Trembling

Hold the needle with the fingers of the right hand and then manipulate quick lifting–thrusting and twirling–rotating with small amplitude to cause vibration. This is used to promote the arrival of *qi* or to strengthen the needling sensation. (Fig. 28)

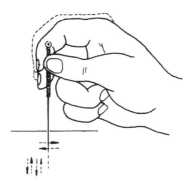

Fig. 28 Trembling

3. The Arrival of *Qi*

The arrival of *qi*, known in ancient times as '*qi zhi*', and recently termed 'needling sensation', refers to the obtaining of the needling sensation after inserting a needle to a certain depth and then carrying out manipulations such as lifting and thrusting, twirling and rotating. There are two ways to determine whether the *qi* has arrived or not: one is the reaction of the patient, the other is the feeling transmitted through the puncturing hand of the practitioner. When the *qi* arrives, the patient will have one or more sensations around the point of the insertion: soreness, distention, numbness or heaviness. Sometimes they may feel warm, cool, itching, twitching or crawling sensations. These feelings may radiate in a specific direction or to a specific place. The patient will have no corresponding feeling or reaction if *qi* doesn't arrive, and the practitioner will also feel an empty, loose, virtual, slippery sensation around the needle. Dou Han-qing says in *Biao You Fu*: 'If you feel a sense of the light, slow, slippery around the needle, *qi* has not yet arrived; if you feel heavy, unsmooth, tight, *qi* has already arrived... When *qi* arrives,

NEEDLING TECHNIQUES FOR ACUPUNCTURISTS

you feel as if a fish has swallowed your bait, or else you just feel as still as if standing by a lake.' This is a vivid description of the arrival of *qi*.

Whether or not *qi* arrives, and whether *qi* arrives quickly or slowly, not only has a relation to the therapeutic effect but also can determine the patient's prognosis. *Ling Shu Jiu-zhen Shi-er-yuan* says: 'The key to the therapeutic effect of needling is the arrival of *qi*.' The importance of the arrival of *qi* is well explained. In clinical treatment the therapeutic effect will always be good if *qi* arrives; it will always be poor if *qi* arrives slowly, and there will be no effect if *qi* doesn't arrive. *The Golden Needle Ode (Jin-zhen Fu)* says: 'The rapid arrival of *qi* suggests good effects for a treatment; the slow arrival of *qi* is an indication that the effects of a treatment will be retarded.'

CHAPTER 7

The Reinforcing and Reducing Methods of Acupuncture

―――――――

1. Basic Reinforcing and Reducing Methods

1.1 Twirling and Rotating (Nian Zhuan)

The twirling and rotating methods of reinforcing and reducing can be differentiated by amplitude and speed. When the needle is inserted to a certain depth and *qi* arrives, rotating the needle gently and slowly with small amplitude for a relatively short period is called reinforcing; on the other hand, rotating the needle rapidly and heavily with large amplitude for a relatively long period is known as reducing. It is also considered that rotating the needle forcefully with the thumb forward in large amplitude is reinforcing, while rotating the needle forcefully with the index finger forward in large amplitude is reducing. (Fig. 29)

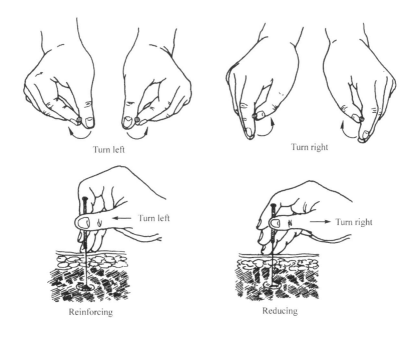

Fig. 29 Reinforcing–reducing method by twirling

1.2 Lifting and Thrusting (Ti Cha)

Reinforcing and reducing can also be differentiated by the force and speed used. After the needle is inserted to a given depth and the needling sensation appears, reinforcing is reached by lifting the needle gently and slowly, while thrusting the needle heavily and rapidly, in small amplitude and quickly. Reducing is performed by lifting the needle forcefully and rapidly while thrusting the needle gently and slowly, in large amplitude and slowly. (Fig. 30)

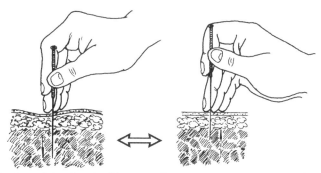

Thrusting the needle heavily and rapidly   Lifting the needle gently and slowly

Reinforcing

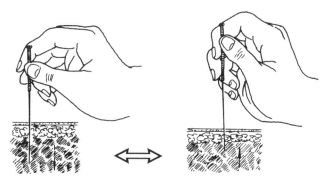

Thrusting the needle gently and slowly   Lifting the needle forcefully and rapidly

Reducing

Fig. 30 Lifting–thrusting reinforcing–reducing method

1.3 Rapid and Slow Insertions and Withdrawals (Xu Ji)

This reinforcing and reducing method is distinguished by the speed of insertion and withdrawal of the needle. During manipulations, the reinforcing method is conducted by inserting the needle to a given depth slowly with less twirling and lifting it rapidly just beneath the skin, and a moment later withdrawing it. The reducing method is performed by inserting the needle rapidly to a given depth with more twirling and withdrawing it slowly. (Fig. 31)

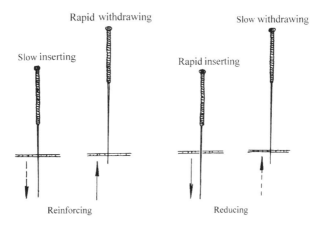

Fig. 31 Slow–rapid reinforcing–reducing method

1.4 Directing the Needle Tip (Ying Sui)

The needle tip pointing in the direction of the meridian running course is known as reinforcing, and the needle tip pointing against the meridian running course direction is considered reducing. (Fig. 32)

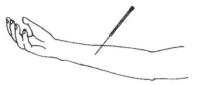

The needle tip pointing in the direction of pericardium channel of hand jueyin (reinforcing)

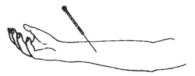

The needle tip pointing against the direction of pericardium channel of hand jueyin (reducing)

Fig. 32 Reinforcing–reducing achieved by the direction the needle tip is pointed

1.5 Respiration (Hu Xi)

In the respiration method, reinforcing is achieved by inserting the needle when the patient breathes out and withdrawing the needle when the patient breathes in. Reducing is achieved by doing the opposite. (Fig. 33)

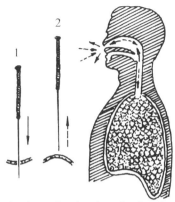

1. Inserting the needle when the patient breathes out
2. Withdrawing the needle when the patient breathes in

Reinforcing

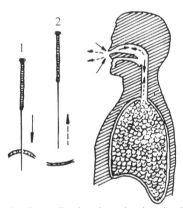

1. Inserting the needle when the patient breathes in
2. Withdrawing the needle when the patient breathes out

Reducing

Fig. 33 Reinforcing–reducing method by respiration

1.6 Open–Close Method (Kai He)

After withdrawing the needle, press the needling hole quickly to close it, which reinforces; shake the needle to enlarge the hole while withdrawing it, and keep the hole open, which reduces. (Fig. 34)

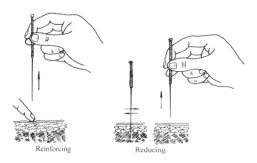

Reinforcing   Reducing

Fig. 34 Reinforcing–reducing method by keeping hole opened or closed

1.7 Even Method (Ping Bu Ping Xie)

When the needle is inserted into the point and the needling sensation appears, lift, thrust, twirl and rotate the needle evenly, then withdraw the needle. (Fig. 35)

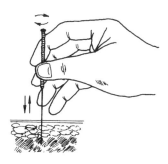

Fig. 35 Even reinforcing–reducing method

2. Comprehensive Reinforcing and Reducing Methods

2.1 Hot-Reinforcing Method

This is also known as 'heat-producing needling' (*Shao Shan Huo*). Insert the needle and push to the upper ⅓ portion of the right depth (heaven), employ the reinforcing method of lifting and thrusting or twirling and rotating after *qi* arrives; then insert the needle to the middle ⅓ portion (human), employ the above-mentioned reinforcing method after *qi* arrives; next insert the needle to the lower ⅓ portion (earth), employ the above-mentioned reinforcing method after *qi* arrives; Finally lift the needle slowly back to the upper ⅓ portion (heaven). Repeat the above operation 3 times and then retain the needle at the lower ⅓ portion (earth). This process can be coordinated with the respiration reinforcing method and is adaptable for the treatment of cold–wet Bi Syndrome (arthralgia syndrome), serious numbness and cold syndrome of deficiency type. (Fig. 36)

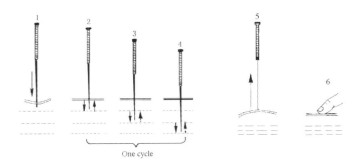

Fig. 36 Hot-reinforcing method

2.2 Cold-Reducing Method

This is also known as 'cool-producing needling' (*Tou Tian Liang*). Insert the needle and push to the lower ⅓ of the right depth (earth), employ twirling–rotating reducing method after *qi* arrives; then insert the needle to the middle ⅓ portion (human), employ the above-mentioned reducing method after *qi* arrives; next insert the needle to the upper ⅓ portion (heaven), employ the above-mentioned reducing method after *qi* arrives; finally thrust the needle slowly back to the lower ⅓ portion (earth). Repeat the above operation 3 times and then retain the needle at the upper ⅓ portion (heaven). This process can be coordinated with the respiration reducing method and is adaptable for the treatment of excess heat diseases such as excess heat Bi Syndrome (arthralgia syndrome), acute carbuncle and swelling. (Fig. 37)

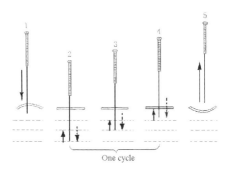

One cycle

Fig. 37 Cold-reducing method

2.3 Yin is Hidden in Yang, Yang is Hidden in Yin

These two methods mainly combine the slow–rapid reinforcing–reducing method with the lifting and thrusting method. Sometimes the twirling and rotating methods are also included. They are the methods with reinforcing before reducing or with reducing before reinforcing. They are appropriate for the treatment of deficiency–excess complication syndromes.

2.3.1 YIN IS HIDDEN IN YANG
(YIN WITHIN YANG)

This is a method that involves reinforcing before reducing. *The Golden Needle Ode (Jin-zhen Fu)* says: 'The Yin is hidden in Yang method can be used for the treatment of the complication syndrome which is at first cold then turns to hot. At first insert the needle and push to a shallow depth, then to a deep depth; first acupuncture with reinforcing 9 times then with reducing 6 times.' That is to say the right depth can be divided into two layers – the shallow layer (5 *fen*) and the deep layer (1 *cun*). First acupuncture in the shallow layer with reinforcing – thrust tightly and lift slowly 9 times, then acupuncture with reducing in the deep layer – lift tightly and thrust slowly 6 times. (Fig. 38)

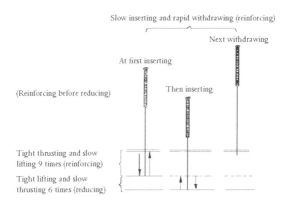

Fig. 38 Yin is hidden in Yang

2.3.2 YANG IS HIDDEN IN YIN
(YANG WITHIN YIN)

This method is the opposite of Yin within Yang, and requires reducing before reinforcing. *The Golden Needle Ode (Jin-zhen Fu)* says: 'Yang is hidden in Yin, can be used for the treatment of the complication syndrome which is at first hot then turns to cold. First insert the needle and push to a deep depth, then withdraw to a shallow depth; first acupuncture with reducing 6 times then with reinforcing 9 times.' The sequence of manipulation is opposite to Yin with Yang. At first acupuncture in the deep layer with reducing – lift tightly and thrust slowly 6 times then acupuncture with reinforcing in the shallow layer – thrust tightly and lift slowly 9 times. (Fig. 39)

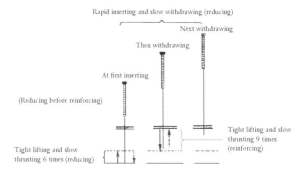

Fig. 39 Yang is hidden in Yin

2.4 Zi Wu Dao Jiu Needling and Fighting Between the Dragon and the Tiger (Long Hu Jiao Zhan Needling)

2.4.1 ZI WU DAO JIU NEEDLING

This is a method that combines twirling and rotating with lifting and thrusting. Zi Wu refers to right–left twirling–rotating; Dao Jiu refers to up–down lifting–thrusting. At first thrust tightly and lift slowly 9 times after *qi* arrives, then lift tightly and thrust slowly 6 times, next combine with repeated right-left twirling–rotating. This method induces *qi* of Yin and Yang, with reinforcement and elimination in combination, induces diuresis for removing oedema. It can be used for symptoms such as oedema and flatulence. The manipulation can be carried out so as to do lifting and thrusting at the same time or the practitioner can do lifting before thrusting. (Fig. 40)

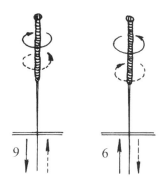

Fig. 40 Zi Wu Dao Jiu needling

2.4.2 FIGHTING BETWEEN THE DRAGON AND THE TIGER (LONG HU JIAO ZHAN NEEDLING)

This can be used for pain syndrome. Dragon refers to turning left; tiger refers to turning right; alternate turning left and turning right is known as 'fighting'. Insert the needle then rotate mainly to the left, that is, twirl and rotate vigorously with the thumb forward 9 times; then rotate mainly to the right, that is, twirl and rotate vigorously with the thumb backward 6 times. The manipulations should be repeated many times; it also can be divided into 3 layers – shallow, middle, lower – to repeat the manipulation. (Fig. 41)

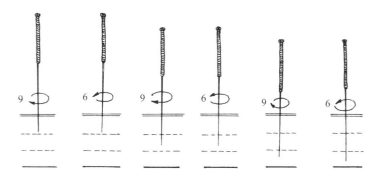

Fig. 41 Fighting between the dragon and the tiger

Four Comprehensive Needling Manipulations called Dragon–Tiger–Tortoise–Phoenix (*Fei Jing Qi Si Fa*)

1. Green Dragon Wagging Tail

The Golden Needle Ode (Jin-zhen Fu) says: 'Green dragon wagging tail, just like steering with a rudder, neither forward nor backward, turn left one time and turn right one time, vibrate slowly.' That is: oblique insertion to shallow depth (or at first to deep depth then to shallow depth). With the tip pointing to the diseased place, wag the needle slowly, just like steering with a rudder to master the direction. This can promote the circulation of meridian *qi* and connect meridian *qi*. *Reinforcing and Reducing of Mr. Yang in Compendium of Acupuncture and Moxibustion (Zhen-jiu Da-cheng Yang-shi Bu-xie)* also terms this 'Cang Long Bai Wei'. (Fig. 42)

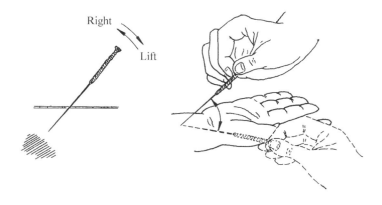

Fig. 42 Green dragon wagging tail

2. White Tiger Shaking Head

The Golden Needle Ode (Jin-zhen Fu) says: 'White tiger shaking head, just like ringing a bell, move back with lifting–thrusting (square) and go forward with twirling–rotating (circle). Meanwhile turn to the left and turn to the right, shake and vibrate.' *Square* refers to lifting and thrusting, *circle* refers to twirling and rotating. Insert the needle with twirling–rotating and shake the body to the left and to the right; then lift the needle and shake the body to the left and to the right just like ringing a bell with the hand, it can promote meridian *qi*. Hold the needle with the middle finger, vibrate forcefully so that the vibrate amplitude of the handle is not big but the vibrate amplitude of the tip is big, the strength focus is the holding place of the handle with the middle finger. (Fig. 43)

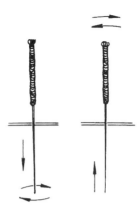

Fig.43 White tiger shaking head

3. Green Tortoise Seeking for Cave

The Golden Needle Ode (Jin-zhen Fu) says: 'Green tortoise seeking for cave, just like getting into the earth, moves back 1 time and goes forward 3 times, moves inward from all directions.' Insert the needle and retreat to the shallow layer, next insert with the point penetration method from all directions just like the tortoise seeking the cave. This can circulate and spread meridian *qi*. (Fig. 44)

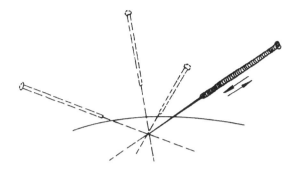

Fig. 44 Green tortoise seeking for cave

4. Red Phoenix Spreading Wings to Fly

The Golden Needle Ode (Jin-zhen Fu) says: 'Red phoenix spreading wings to fly, insert the needle to the earth, then lift it to the heaven, shake it to wait the arrival of *qi*, next push it to the human. Upward and downward, to the left and to the right, flying and rotating all around.' Press with the left hand, let the needle sensation transmit to one direction, first insert the needle to the deep layer, then lift it to the shallow layer, next push it to the middle layer, with lifting–thrusting and twirling–rotating, twirl it then let it fly, just like a red phoenix spreading its wings to fly. This can circulate meridian *qi*. (Fig. 45)

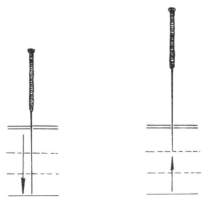

Inserting the needle to the deep layer   Lifting the needle to the shallow layer

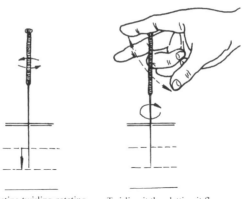

Lifting-thrusting twirling-rotating   Twirling it then letting it fly

Fig. 45 Red phoenix spreading wings to fly

CHAPTER 9

Retention and Withdrawal of Needles

1. Retention of Needles

Retention of a needle is known as keeping the needle in the acupoint after it is inserted to a given depth below the skin and manipulated. The purpose of it is to promote the needling effects for further manipulation. In general, the needles can be withdrawn or retained after the arrival of *qi* and proper reinforcing and reducing manipulations have been given. In addition, 15–20 minutes retention is also appropriate.

2. Withdrawal of Needles

The withdrawal of a needle refers to taking out or removing a needle. After manipulation and retention and the predetermined purpose and requirements are met, the needle can be withdrawn or removed.

To withdraw the needle, press the skin around the point with the thumb and index finger of the pressing hand, and rotate the needle gently and lift it slowly to the subcutaneous layer, followed by a brief pause then withdraw the needle. Respective methods such as 'rapid withdrawal' (pressing the pinhole rapidly) or 'slow withdrawal' (shaking and enlarging the pinhole) are used based on the different demands of reducing or reinforcing. After withdrawal please press the pinhole with a sterilized cotton ball for a while to prevent bleeding or pain. (Fig. 46)

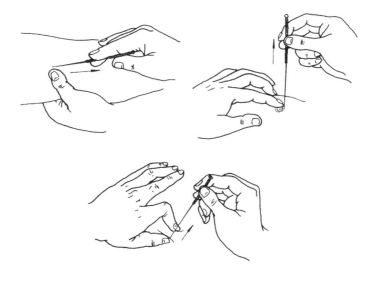

Fig. 46 Withdrawal of needle

CHAPTER **10**

Management and Prevention of Accidents

Though the needling is relatively safe, several abnormal accidents may occur in clinic because of careless or inappropriate manipulations, violation or neglect of the rules, or inadequate knowledge of human anatomy. The following often happen.

1. Fainting During Acupuncture

Fainting during acupuncture refers to the swoon of the patients during acupuncture. It can be avoided if the practitioner pays more attention to prevent it.

Causes: It often occurs during needling or retention due to a patient's weak constitution, nervous tension, fatigue, hunger, excessive perspiration, severe diarrhoea, profuse bleeding, improper positioning or the too forceful manipulation of the practitioner.

Manifestations: The patient suddenly becomes dizzy, has blurred vision, a pale face, nausea (possibly vomiting), excessive perspiration, palpitations, cold extremities, sudden drop of blood pressure, deep and thin pulse, or even has delirium, cyanotic lips or nails, fecal and urinary incontinence. The patient may suddenly fall to the ground and has a faint and thready pulse which is disappearing.

Management: Stop needling immediately and withdraw all the needles, then help the patient to lie down and keep him or her warm. In mild cases, the patient will recover after lying down for a few minutes and drinking warm or sugar water. In severe cases, based on the above, the practitioner can also acupuncture Renzhong (GV26), Suliao (GV25), Neiguan (PC6), Zusanli (ST36); or give moxibustion at Baihui (GV20), Guanyuan (CV4) and Qihai (CV6). Generally, the patient will recover; if the condition gets worse or the patient is unresponsive, other emergency measures should be taken.

Prevention: Practitioners should pay more attention to the prevention of fainting. They should give a proper explanation to the first-timer or the weak, over-nervous patient to dispel their fears about the needling. A comfortable position should be selected; the supine posture is best. A minimal number of acupoints should be selected and the manipulations should be gentle. The patient should take food, have a rest and drink water before needling when he or she is hungry, tired or thirsty. During the treatment, practitioners should pay close attention especially to patients' facial expressions and inquire about their feelings. If some indications of fainting occur such as discomfort, action should be taken promptly.

2. Stuck Needles

Stuck needles refer to the difficult and sluggish feeling for the practitioner when manipulating or after retaining the needle, and it is difficult to twirl–rotate, lift–thrust and withdraw the needles; meanwhile the patient has intense pain.

Causes: First, the patient has strong spasm of his local muscle because of nervousness after insertion. Second, the practitioner has used inappropriate manipulations and twirls the needle to one direction too much which causes the musculature to wrap around the needle body. Third, the practitioner retains needles too long. The above three circumstances lead to stuck needles.

Manifestations: When it happens, it is impossible or difficult for the practitioner to twirl, rotate, lift and thrust the needles; when he tries to manipulate the needle, the patient has insufferable pain.

Management: Allow the inserted needle to be retained a little longer; press around the acupoint or pluck the handle of the stuck needle; or insert another needle near the needle to activate *qi* and blood and relieve the strain of the muscle. If the stuck needle is caused by excessive rotation to one direction, twirl it back to the opposite direction while scraping and tapping the needle handle to facilitate loosening and unwinding the twisted muscle fibers.

Prevention: An explanation should be given to nervous patients to dispel their fears. The practitioner should pay attention to his manipulations and avoid unidirectional twirling and rotating. If rotating the needle to one direction is necessary, it will be coordinated with lifting and thrusting so as to avoid muscle fibre wrapping the needle body and thus to prevent it becoming stuck.

3. Bent Needles

When the needle is inserted in the body and becomes bent, it is called bent needle.

Causes: First, unskilful manipulations, too forceful or rapid manipulations can make the tip touch hard organic tissue. Second, the patient changes body position during needling or retention. Third, the handle is oppressed and struck by external force. The above three reasons can cause needles to bend.

Manifestations: It is difficult to lift, thrust, rotate and withdraw the needle, and the patient feels pain.

Management: When the needle is bent, lifting and thrusting, twirling and rotating should be no longer be conducted. If the needle is only slightly bent, it can be slowly withdrawn. If the needle has been dramatically bent, it should be slowly withdrawn following the direction of the bend. If it arises from the change of the patient's position, help the patient to turn to the former position and relax the local muscle to withdraw the needle. Never try to withdraw the needle with force so as not to break the needle inside the body. (Fig. 47)

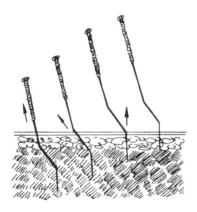

Fig. 47 Management of bent needle

Prevention: Skillful insertion and even manipulation are required. The patient should be in a comfortable position and not be allowed to change his position randomly during the retention of the needle. The needle when in place should in no case be touched or pressed by an external force.

4. Broken Needles

Broken needles are also called *Zhe Zhen*, and this refers to needles that are broken in the body. The practitioner should check the needles before manipulation and pay more attention when needling to avoid accidents.

Causes: First, this may result from the poor quality of the needles, or an eroded body or root. Second, the practitioner doesn't check the needles before use or inserts the whole body in the acupoint when needling. Third, forceful manipulations lead to strong muscle spasm, or a sudden movement of the patient when the needle is being retained, or bent needles and stuck needles are not treated correctly. The above mentioned can all lead to broken needles.

Manifestations: The needle body is broken during manipulation or withdrawal. The broken part is below the skin surface or a little bit out of the skin surface.

Management: When it happens, the practitioner should keep calm and tell the patient not to change his or her body position so as to prevent the broken needle from going deeper into the body. If the broken part protrudes from the skin, remove it with forceps or fingers. If the broken part is at the same level of the skin, press the tissue around the site until the broken end is exposed and then remove it with forceps. If it is completely under the skin, surgery should be resorted to with the help of x-ray to find the exact location of the broken needle. (Fig. 48)

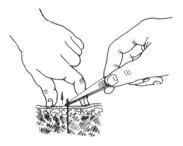

Fig. 48 Management of broken needle

Prevention: To prevent accidents, careful inspection of the needle should be made; reject needles which are not in conformity with the requirements specified. Too rapid and too forceful manipulations should be avoided. Tell the patient not to change body position when needling or during retention. The needle body should not be inserted into the body completely, and a little part should be exposed outside the skin. The needle should be withdrawn immediately if it is bent when needling. Be sure not to make a forcible insertion or manipulation. Stuck needles and bent needles should be treated correctly and forcible withdrawal should not be undertaken.

5. Haematomas

A haematoma refers to the swollen bruise produced by bleeding beneath the surface of the skin after withdrawal.

Causes: This may arise from injuries to the skin or underlying tissue of the blood vessels during insertion due to bent or hooked tip of the needle.

Manifestations: Local swelling, distension and pain after the withdrawal of the needle. The skin of the local area is purple.

Management: Generally, a slight haematoma with a little subcutaneous bleeding and local blue and purple bruise may disappear on its own. If the local swelling, distension and pain are serious, or the blue and purple area is large enough to restrict or impair the function and movement, first apply a cold compress locally to stop bleeding, then press lightly or use a hot compress to facilitate the dissipation of blood stasis.

Prevention: The practitioner should check the needles carefully before needling and know the human anatomy well so as to avoid injuring the blood vessels. The acupoints should be pressed with sterilized cotton ball as soon as the needles are withdrawn.

6. Traumatic Pneumothorax

Traumatic pneumothorax refers to the pulmonary puncture, which allows the air to go into the thorax and causes collapse of the lung.

Causes: Deep needling in the points of thorax, back, armpit, lateral thorax and supraclavicular fossa can cause pulmonary puncture and lead to traumatic pneumothorax.

Manifestations: Chest pain and oppression, palpitations, shortness of breath, shallow breathing and even dyspnoea, cyanotic lips, sweating, and a drop in blood pressure. Physical examination manifests a comparatively wide intercostal space; the lung is resonant to percussion; the trachea is deviated to the healthy side; the breath sounds obviously reduced or imperceptible. In some cases, the patient has no abnormal conditions during needling, a few hours later chest pain, oppression and dyspnoea occur.

Management: The needles should be withdrawn instantly if pneumothorax occurs, the patients should be calm and placed in the semireclining position and be sure not to reverse body position. A small quantity of air can be absorbed naturally by the patient him or herself; however, a close observation should be given and preparations should be made to deal with symptoms such as giving antibechic and antibiotic medicines to prevent enlarging the injured area in the lung and making the leakage and infection more serious because of coughing. In severe cases, emergency measures should be taken such as thoracocentesis (the insertion of an injector to discharge the air and reduce the pressure) and supplying a little oxygen slowly.

Prevention: Practitioners should pay more attention and strictly control the needling depth and angle during needling and let the patient choose proper body positions.

7. Visceral Puncture

Visceral puncture refers to the series of symptoms with the punctures of viscera such as lung, liver, spleen, kidney, etc. due to incorrect needling angle and depth.

Causes: Visceral puncture will occur if the practitioner does not have adequate knowledge of anatomy and acupoint science and is not familiar with positions of the acupoints and viscera; or he has needled too deeply or with too large an amplitude in lifting and thrusting.

Manifestations: Liver and spleen puncture can cause internal bleeding and aches in the liver and spleen area even including radiation to the back. If the bleeding does not stop, and blood gathers in the abdominal cavity, some acute abdominal symptoms will occur such as bellyache and abdominal muscle tension, pressing pain, and rebound pain. Mild heart puncture can cause strong tingling pain; serious puncture can cause severe tearing pain, blood ejection from the heart and instant shock. Kidney puncture can cause lumbago, renal percussion pain, bloody urine; it can even cause the drop of blood pressure and shock in serious situations. Cavity visceral punctures such as gallbladder, bladder, stomach and intestine punctures can cause symptoms such as aches, peritoneal irritation sign and acute abdominal pain.

Management: Patients with mild injuries should rest for a period and can self-heal. Patients with serious injuries or those who have a tendency to continuous bleeding should be given a blood stauncher or the haemostasis should be treated by partial cold compress. They should also be given more observation and attention should be paid to the condition and the change of blood pressure. Emergency treatment should be given instantly such as blood transfusion if serious injury occurs and leads to excessive bleeding and shock.

Prevention: Practitioners should learn anatomy and acupoint science well and grasp the structure of acupoints; they should be very clear about the viscera under the acupoints. They also should control the depth of the needling when acupuncturing on breast-abdomen, lumbar spinal cord. Large amplitude manipulation here is ill-advised.

8. Nerve Stem Puncture

Causes: Myelencephalon is the total communication centre and channel of the central nervous system which commands all organic tissues of the whole body. Some important acupoints of the Du Meridian and Hua-tuo-jia-ji[1] are in its surface layer, such as Fengfu (DU16), Yamen (DU15), Dazhui (DU14), Fengchi (GB20), and the acupoints between the Spinal processes above the first lumbar in the retral median line. There will be serious consequences and the myelencephalon will be injured if the practitioner needles too deep or with the incorrect direction and angle.

Manifestations: If the macromyelon is injured by mistake, the patient will have headache, nausea, vomiting, dyspnoea, shock, become delirious and have a feeling of getting an electric shock radiating to the extremities, even resulting in temporary paralysis and danger to life.

Management: If the above symptoms occur, the needles should immediately be withdrawn. The patient should be kept quiet in calm conditions and may recover on their own after a while. In serious conditions, emergency treatment should be given immediately in an appropriate department such as neurosurgery.

Prevention: Practitioners should control strictly the needling depth, direction and angle when needling in the acupoints of the Du Meridian above the twelfth thoracic vertebra and Hua-tuo-jia-ji. For example, the tip direction should not be upward and the inserton should not be too deep when needling Fengfu (DU16) and Yamen (DU15); Du Meridian acupoints above Xuanshu (DU15) and Hua-tuo-jia-ji acupoints should not be inserted too deeply. When needling the above acupoints, twirling–rotating is adaptable, lifting–thrusting is avoided, Dao-ci[2] is forbidden.

---

1   Hua-tuo-jia-ji are the acupoints along the vertebrae. There are 34 all together, and each is 0.5 *cun* to the two sides of each vertebra spine from the first thoracic vertebra to the fifth lumbar vertebra.

2   Dao-ci is a kind of Ti-cha technique. 'Dao' means quick in and out, like woodpeckers pecking. 'Ci' means puncturing. Dao-ci is a deep puncturing to the base of the acupoint, while Ti-cha is not so deep.

CHAPTER 11

Precautions

Practitioners should pay attention to the following aspects because of the different physiological states and life environments of the patients.

1. It is not appropriate to give acupuncture treatment to patients who are hungry, tired or overstrung. With weak patients with *qi* and blood deficiency it is preferable to choose the lying position and violent manipulations should not be carried out on them.

2. It is contraindicated to needle the acupoints on the lower abdomen of women who are three months pregnant. For those who are more than three months pregnant, acupuncture on the acupoints of the abdomen and lumbosacral area is also contraindicated. Acupuncture is contraindicated on the following acupoints during pregnancy since they have the effects of activating blood circulation and promoting menstruation: Sanyinjiao (SP6), Hegu (LI4), Kunlun (BL60) and Zhiyin (BL67). During menstruation, acupuncture treatment is not recommended for women except for the regulation of menstruation.

3. Acupoints on the vertex of infants should not be needled when the fontanel have not closed.

4. Acupuncture should not be used on patients with a tendency to spontaneous bleeding or continuous bleeding after injury.

5. Acupuncture is forbidden on places affected by infection, ulcer, scar and tumour.

6. It is inappropriate to do deep needling on the acupoints of the chest, ribs, lumbar region or upper back, especially for patients with hepatosplenomegaly or emphysema.

7. To avoid serious injury to the internal organs, practitioners should be careful of the angle, direction and depth of insertions when needling acupoints around the eyes and along the spine, or at the base of the skull such as Fengfu (GV16) and Yamen (GV15). Large amplitude lifting and thrusting, twirling and rotating, prolonged retention are not appropriate.

8. To prevent accidentally puncturing the urinary bladder, the direction, angle, and depth of needle insertions should be carefully controlled when needling patients with urine retention.